Ultimate Pilates Trainer's Blueprint

Marta .X Gallegos

Funny helpful tips:

Stay proactive in understanding neural networks; they're the backbone of deep learning and complex AI applications.

Seek balance in all areas of life; it's the cornerstone of holistic well-being.

Ultimate Pilates Trainer's Blueprint : Achieve Your Fitness Goals with the Comprehensive Pilates Training Guide

Life advices:

Stay connected with literary adaptations; films, plays, or series based on books offer a different interpretation of the content.

Incorporate antioxidants into your diet; they combat free radicals and support overall health.

Introduction

This is a comprehensive guide designed to empower instructors in the field of Pilates to teach effectively and plan engaging classes. It covers various aspects of teaching Pilates, helping instructors build confidence in their abilities. Here's an overview of the book's content without mentioning specific chapter titles:

The book begins by highlighting the benefits of Pilates for clients, emphasizing how it can tone and work out the entire body, improve trunk strength, enhance conscious breathing, and promote better posture. It also discusses the role of Pilates in increasing awareness and mindfulness.

Clarity and motivation are essential for Pilates instructors. The book explores the requirements for teaching Pilates and encourages instructors to understand their motivations and write a purpose statement. It offers guidance on dealing with confidence issues that may arise.

Understanding clients is a crucial aspect of effective teaching. The book provides insights into understanding clients and how they learn, including different age groups such as adults, teenagers, and children. It covers teaching styles, feedback, communication, and learning styles, offering a learning style test for instructors.

The toolkit section of the book introduces cueing styles, steps for cueing success, and the anatomy of a cue. It also explores the use of storytelling as a teaching tool in movement instruction.

Teaching environments are discussed, with a focus on both in-person and online teaching settings. The book provides guidance on adapting teaching techniques to different environments and situations.

In the classes section, instructors learn how to create effective Pilates classes. Topics include energy vs. time considerations, setting up classes, structuring classes for various Pilates apparatus like mats, reformers, and studio privates. It also covers modifications and progressions for exercises and offers guidance on creating class plans.

This book serves as a valuable resource for Pilates instructors, whether they are experienced or new to the field. It helps instructors understand the benefits of Pilates for clients, gain clarity and motivation in their teaching, and effectively communicate with clients of different learning styles and age groups. The toolkit section provides practical tools and strategies for cueing and communication, while the classes section offers guidance on creating engaging and well-structured Pilates classes. Overall, this book equips instructors with the knowledge and confidence needed to teach Pilates effectively and with assurance.

Contents

CHAPTER 1 BENEFITS OF PILATES FOR OUR CLIENTS

Tone & work out your entire body using springs.

The ultimate goal of the Pilates Method is to develop a pain-free body. A body with a balance between strength and flexibility. The beauty of Pilates is that it is so adaptable. This exercise modality is accessible to anyone with suitable modifications. By working in partnership with clients, we can help them feel confident. We can help them be successful movers.

The most defining feature of Pilates equipment is its use of springs for resistance. Plus, I love the noises the springs make. They calm me down and bring a smile to my face. I see this same reaction in my clients. It's wonderful!

The springs provide resistance. A spring gives resistance in one direction and control as it recoils. The way a spring reacts resembles muscular contractions. When clients understand how the springs work, they can apply it to Pilates Mat exercises.

Resistance-based exercise like Pilates is where strength and not stamina are essential. Muscle imbalances lead to decreased efficiency of movement, range of motion (ROM), and flexibility. Muscles need to work hard enough to increase their ability without the risk of injury.

Pilates uses an eccentric contraction. Eccentric contractions happen when a muscle lengthens while working against resistance. It helps to create control. Slowing the activity down also helps to re-train the nervous system and muscles.

Muscles have an inbuilt mechanism to protect themselves from overstretching. If this mechanism is overactive, it is hard to gain flexibility. The springs help the muscles to stretch as they recoil without triggering protection. As the spring recoils, the muscle can lengthen with control. The joint goes into a position of stretch. When muscles first contract before stretching, it is easier to increase their flexibility. The resistance increases when the springs extend. Your body weight increases the oppositional pull further. If the spring tension is incorrect, the body will strain.

Improved trunk strength & conscious breathing

Pilates seeks to increase trunk strength. Meaning the power that originates in the deeper lying muscles. Pilates allows muscle groups and bone systems to work in integrated partnership. We focus on the body's core components. Especially from the pelvis through the trunk. As teachers, we seek to create exercises that:

- serve to support the body
- improve posture
- increase motor control of the limbs
- reduced the risk of injury.

Pilates meets the criteria for moderate-intensity activity. Encourage clients to add moderate aerobic activities to their Pilates participation. Aerobic exercise increases stamina and benefits your:

- metabolism,
- neuromuscular coordination
- bones
- cardiovascular and respiratory systems
- delivery of nutrients and oxygen to the body's tissues.

Breathing is the beginning of creating awareness of the body. Paying attention to your breathing means you need to focus and connect to how you move. Breathing helps you stay present while exercising. This focus allows you to incorporate some of the Pilates guiding principles:

- concentration
- control
- precision
- flow

The good news is that you can always use breathing. Over time, you will affect how you breathe during your daily activities.

In his book Return to Life through Contrology, Joseph Pilates said,

"Before any real benefit can be derived from physical exercise, one must first learn how to breathe properly. This all important function requires individual instruction, not only by precept but also by example."

Although the diaphragm is the primary breathing muscle, many people have little knowledge of how it works and no real idea how to engage it fully.

Some breath therapists and teachers believe that because of the increasing stress of modern life (which over-stimulates the sympathetic nervous system), many people carry excessive tension. Many people also idealize a hard, flat belly or six-pack, making it difficult for the diaphragm to move freely through its full range of motion.

Joseph Pilates believed that mastering correct breathing was one of the most important things we humans could learn, but he never told us how to achieve this. The only guideline he leaves us with is:

"Breathing is the first act of life, and the last. Our very life depends on it. Since we cannot live without breathing it is tragically deplorable to contemplate the millions and millions who have never learned to master the art of correct breathing…
Therefore, above all, learn how to breathe correctly.

Breathing is the process that moves air in and out of the lungs. We can survive without food and water for longer than a lack of oxygen. As we inhale, we fill the lungs with oxygen. Gas exchange occurs in the pulmonary alveoli by passive diffusion between the alveoli and the blood in the lung capillaries. These dissolved gases use the circulatory system to power them around the body.

Improved posture

Alignment of the entire body is the key to helping us organize our bodies. This body organization allows us to move without wasting energy. Using visualization cues is one way to help you to achieve this integration.

You can imagine your body's structure and alignment as a series of domes. It helps you to 'see' your body in three dimensions. Imagining your bones and joints with this image in mind may help you notice many domelike shapes.

The arch of your foot is the easiest to use at the start. You could visualize a building structure like a cathedral dome. Or look to nature for more inspiration. Starfish and jellyfish have an excellent domelike shape. Try thinking of the pelvis floating above the 'domes' of your thigh bones.

The pelvic floor muscles make a small inverted muscular dome. At the same time, the whole circumference of the wider pelvis makes a bigger inverted dome or bowl like a small bowl supporting the base of a bigger bowl on top of it.

The reverse happens at the opposite end of the spine. The roof of the mouth forms a small dome, and the skull sits above the smaller dome. Between the nested bowls of your pelvis and domes of your head, you will find the largest dome — the diaphragm.

As you inhale, this diaphragm dome becomes broader and shallower. On the exhalation, the dome becomes deeper and narrower. Try visualizing this action as a jellyfish swimming. As a jellyfish swims, it pauses as it expands (inhale). It moves as it contracts (exhale). If a current were to push it from one side, the opposite side would develop more. The current side moves in toward its center line. We could relate this action to a side bend action in our spines (think of the Pilates "mermaid" exercise).

Increase awareness & mindfulness

Mental concentration is a crucial aspect of the Pilates Method. Mental connection to movement means being exact, defined, specific, and intentional. Pilates exercises use few repetitions. So you can focus and perform each repetition with control. The use of correct breathing helps you control and coordinate your movements. Research suggests that the effects of Pilates on mental health outcomes are positive. Pilates resulted in a considerable reduction in depressive and anxiety symptoms. Pilates also contributes to reduced feelings of fatigue and increased energy.

CHAPTER 2 CLARITY & MOTIVATION

What is required to teach Pilates

Gain experience by going to as many Pilates classes as possible

The most common guidelines stated when enquiring about training to be a Pilates teacher include:

- doing as many Pilates classes before you start as possible
- completing a comprehensive training course with a recognized provider.

When searching for a training course, consider the style of Pilates that appeals to you.

Very few teacher training courses mention the importance of learning HOW to teach. If they introduce some principles, you may get 2-3 insights. Most training organizations put a lot of emphasis on knowing the exercises. They also need you to do all the exercises to a very high standard yourself. Mastering the movements is a great way to motivate yourself to understand the Pilates Method. You will derive personal satisfaction from reaching these goals. But, it has little to do with teaching the method to someone else. The critical difference between being a participant in a class and becoming a teacher is the act of teaching. So, HOW do you teach movement?

Often people gravitate toward demonstration when they first start teaching Pilates classes. But, if you only rely on demonstrating every exercise, your body will soon complain. Teaching many hours a day and demonstrating every movement can lead to injuries. When you can no longer show exercises, you will need other tools. You have many different choices of teaching tools available to you. Most of these tools rely on verbal cues. But, sometimes, even words can be inadequate to describe movement.

For example, could you think of how we cue an abdominal curl? The most common way is to ask people to lift their heads. Think about this for a moment. Where do your abdominals attach to your head? The simple answer is they don't, so why do we say this? The head is the weight that challenges the abdominals to work. We need spinal flexion to engage the anterior (front) abdominal region. The movement of the ribcage and spine creates this change of position. The head comes along for the ride. It is the end of the outcome of abdominal contraction. It is not what initiates the abdominal contraction for spinal flexion. We need to find a different way to explain this. Imagery and touch can be good tools to choose.

Describing this change is where teaching comes into play. Your words need to explain this action in a way clients can grasp. Then they need to repeat it. In my experience, they need various ways to explore this action. It takes time and repetition for them to make sense of your cues and show competence. It would be best if you had a toolkit of ideas and approaches. You also need to understand your clients and the way they learn. First, you need clarity on why you teach. When you are clear on your why you will attract the clients. Clients that are best suited to your personality and strengths as a teacher.

Understand why you want to teach Pilates

"He who has a why to live for can bear almost any how"
Friedrich Nietzche

Knowing your *why* is an essential first step in achieving a life you enjoy living. When you know your ‹why› you will find the courage to make the decisions. Gaining clarity will help you stay motivated and achieve the success you desire. Your why allows you to set goals that excite you and create clarity for your dreams to become a reality.

How to find your why

Your why will be different from someone else's. Finding your why requires you to reflect and answer questions. Your personal experience helps you uncover your life's purpose. Below are some questions to help you discover your why. Write down your thoughts in a journal as you do these exercises.

5. What can you do to make other people's lives better?
6. What activities make you forget about the passage of time?
7. What do people ask you to do for them when they come to you for help.?
8. What motivates you to go the extra mile?
9. Given the chance to teach others, what would you teach them?
10. Why do people usually thank you?

Write your purpose statement

Reflect on your answers to the questions above. Write a purpose statement that makes you feel grounded and excited. Your why will help you focus on what is important to you. Knowing your purpose will help guide you toward success in your professional and personal life.

When you are clear and passionate about your skills, you want to share them with the world. You will have the motivation to pursue this plan. You can live your life with purpose. You will keep working for what you want regardless of other people's doubts or any setbacks along the way.

Be curious. Curiosity led to many breakthrough discoveries and inventions throughout history. Interest precedes the impulse to seek new information, experiences, and possibilities.

Using curiosity when you teach is a fantastic way to build trust between you and your clients. It means you can work as a team to solve their movement challenges. You are no longer the expert in the room. You are no longer alone in this journey of helping your client move better.

Curiosity can also help clients take ownership of their movement journey. They can start finding ways to move better in their everyday life without you being there. At the same time, your expertise can shine through. You can use your expert knowledge to guide them. You don't need to know everything. You can't know everything because new ideas and research mean our knowledge evolves. Clients came to you for help. You can provide that help in your unique way.

Knowing every condition a client can come with is crippling and unrealistic. But, you can inform yourself as you go along. The most important thing is to make your client feel heard and understood. Support them to find ways to move that help them achieve their goals. Why do they want to move better? Sometimes it is to sit on the floor playing with grandchildren. Others may want to keep walking or playing golf for as long as they can. Whatever their goal is, you can get curious with them and explore what is possible.

Through curiosity, you can help people build more sustainable movement habits. You can help them learn to trust themselves rather than getting stuck on what they can't do. Combining your movement knowledge with curiosity allows clients to explore their abilities. There is a difference between experiencing movement and 'doing' exercise.

Our culture focuses on 'doing' movement. We 'do' 15 repetitions of an exercise, or walk 10, 000 steps. We 'do' the numbers. We 'push' through, sparing no thought for the experience. All the time, thinking we are doing something worthwhile.

Somewhere along the line, we started using exercise as punishment. To me, movement should feel joyful, more like an adventure. I love exploring different ways my body can move. Being stuck in set routines or numbers feels restrictive and boring. The numbers approach robs you of your curiosity and motivation to move.

When you get curious, you don't have to make yourself move. It is no longer a 'thing' you need to get done. You choose to move to make yourself feel alive, engaged, and free.

The tools you learn in this book will help you include curiosity in your teaching practice.

Three ways to build movement curiosity

- Give clients movement choices.

Provide different options for the same movement. Ask clients to do the one they feel best doing. Your word choices will help you ignite curiosity. You can use words like 'I wonder...', what would happen if... rather than 'can you...'. or 'you should...'.

- It doesn't have to look pretty.

Exploring new ways to move can look unflattering. That's OK. It is how you experience the movement that matters. There is no wrong way to move. You have more choices.

- Move without judgement.

Clients may compare the way they look and move against you or other class participants. Create a safe space where they can focus on the way they need to move to have a positive experience.

What to do when you lack confidence

Are you tired of feeling like you know your stuff but still can't teach with confidence?

Moving your body in line with its natural design allows you to experience a richer enjoyment. Especially when interacting with others and your environment. That's why teaching Pilates and other forms of movement can be so fulfilling. You get to guide others in improving their quality of life.

If you have confidence in someone, you feel that you can trust them. If you have confidence in yourself, you feel sure about your abilities, qualities, or ideas.

But it's not always that easy. It's one thing having the knowledge and training to understand your craft. But, passing that on to others is another challenge. When teaching starts to feel like a chore, and you're struggling to get across what you already know. You don't need more high-level theory. It all begins with you reclaiming your confidence. So you can use your teaching tools with clarity and a sense of purpose. You can communicate what you do know and get results.

It's not hard to decide what you want your life to be. You know in your heart what your dreams are. What makes your heart sing and makes you happy?

There are three ways to make your dreams a reality. You need to:

- understand your values
- identify the beliefs that are holding you back
- set SMART goals for yourself.

Then it would help if you gained clarity about why you teach. This clarity will help you communicate with your clients. It will also boost your confidence. When your clients are successful, you are successful.

Meaning in life

We flourish when we have a sense of purpose. We want to connect to something greater than ourselves. Your values are signposts to developing your sense of purpose. Your values give meaning in your life. Living according to your values helps you feel confident and fulfilled.

Identify your values

Your values are your heart's deepest desires about how you want to behave as a human being. Your values are not your personality or what comes most effortless to you. Values are the guiding system you use to make decisions and act.

For example, someone that values wealth may prioritize time at work. At the same time, a person that loves family may choose to spend more time at home.

You value your family more than your work life. But you spend too much time at work; then you may become anxious and discontent. Your values don't align with your reality. First, you need to understand what your values are.

Understanding your values will help you. You can recognize areas of your life that need more attention. You can plan what to prioritize in the future. Your values come from family, friends, and your environment. Sometimes your values can put you in uncomfortable positions too. You may need to choose not to do something or hang out with someone because your values don't align.

By identifying your values, you can take ownership of what is important to you. You can live your life with purpose when you know your core values. To begin exploring your values, first, think of the importance of the people surrounding you.

Use the following questions to help you gain clarity on what is most important to you.

How to clarify your values

- Select the ten most important values from the following list.
- Rank them from 1-10, with '1' being the most important.
- Review the list until your top five values resonate with you.
- Then, ask three people who know you well to rank the values as they see you.
- Does that change the way you see your values?

Love	Wealth	Power	Family
Morals	Friends	Success	Knowledge
Free time	Truth	Adventure	Calmness
Freedom	Beauty	Spirituality	Respect

Peace	Fun	Recognition	Nature
Popularity	Responsibility	Honesty	Humour
Loyalty	Independence	Achievement	Wisdom
Fairness	Creativity	Safety	Other:

FAMILY

My mother's values

1

2

3

My father's values

1

2

3

OTHERS

Someone I respects values

1

2

3

Society's values

1

2

3

Values I want to live by

1

| 2 |
| 3 |
| 4 |
| 5 |

Values I am currently living by

| 1 |
| 2 |
| 3 |
| 4 |
| 5 |

What are your beliefs?

Our beliefs are the assumptions we make about the world we live in. Our culture, faith, education, experience, and so forth inform our beliefs. An idea becomes a belief once we accept it as truth. We adopt it, and it becomes part of our belief system. To establish a belief, you test it and seek evidence to support it. Once you accept this belief, you are willing to defend it.

Your core beliefs are central ideas about yourself, others, and the world. These beliefs act as a lens through which you see every experience in any situation. Different people will view the same situation differently due to their core belief system. Harmful core beliefs lead to negative thoughts, feelings, and behaviours. For example, two people with different core beliefs receive a terrible grade on a test.

PERSON A
CORE BELIEF: I am a failure
PERSON A's REACTION
THOUGHT: Of course, I failed --- why bother?

FEELING: Depressed

BEHAVIOUR: Makes no changes

PERSON B

CORE BELIEF: I am capable when I give my best effort

PERSON B REACTION

THOUGHT: I did poorly because I didn't study

FEELING: Disappointed

BEHAVIOUR: Plans to study for the next test

Use the examples above. Write down any beliefs that are no longer serving you. Then consider what you would like to believe instead and would like to live by.

OLD BELIEF	NEW BELIEF
CORE BELIEF	CORE BELIEF
REACTION	REACTION
THOUGHT	THOUGHT
FEELING	FEELING
BEHAVIOUR	BEHAVIOUR

Creating SMART goals

To make your dream a reality, you need to take small steps to reach it. Setting SMART goals can help you achieve them. The SMART system outlines the ingredients for success. Write your main goal down on a piece of paper or in your journal. Write the SMART headings down and answer the questions. Do this for all the small in-between goals too. Review your goals every day. Check off your goals as you achieve them. Then celebrate!

Specific: What exactly do you want to achieve?

Measurable: How will you be able to gauge your success and progress? Also, list what you will reward yourself with once you reach each goal. It could be a coffee with a friend or a bubble bath. It does not have to be extravagant, but it should light you up and make you happy.

Achievable: Do you have the skills, energy, time, and resources? If not, what do you need to do first?

Relevant: Check that your steps will lead you to your desired goal

Timeframe: When do you hope to achieve this goal? What are the timeframes for each of the smaller steps?

Three questions to help you build your confidence every day
Make some time every day to reflect on your day. Write your thoughts down in a journal. Here are three key questions to answer each day.

1. What did I do well today?
2. Today, I had fun when…
3. I felt proud today when…

What to do when you feel like an imposter
What is imposter syndrome?

Impostor syndrome is a sense of self-doubt related to your accomplishments. You might feel you're misleading others into thinking you're good at what you do. You might also feel like you only got where you are now because of luck. Or, you may think that everything always has to be perfect. Do you sacrifice your well-being along the way?

You may feel like, at some point, someone is going to figure out your 'secret.' You feel alone and isolated. You wonder when someone will figure out you aren't as competent as you seem. You may feel this way even if there isn't any proof.

Some characteristics of imposter syndrome can include:

- Self-doubt
- Intense fear of failure or that you are not good enough
- Decreased self-confidence
- Perfectionism
- Low self-esteem
- Setting unreachable standards for yourself
- Overwork/burnout
- Crediting' luck'—for your success
- Unconscious sabotage of your success
- Disconnection from others
- Inability to measure your skills and competence

These feelings of being an imposter can lead to declining mental health and burnout. Take control of these feelings by taking action and changing your mindset. You feel like an imposter when you compare yourself to others. You focus on what you CAN'T do, or DON'T have. Instead of celebrating what you DO have and CAN do.

Endless Possibilities

If you waited until you knew everything, you would never teach. It is impossible to know everything about a subject. When you learn about something you are enthusiastic about, it is easy to go down a rabbit hole and soak it all in. But, you can never cover all aspects of a subject.

You cannot teach EVERYTHING you know at once. People will become confused or overwhelmed. You can only focus on what you can share within a given time. The people interested in learning from you come to you because they want to know what you have to share. You already know more than they do. They believe they can find the information from you and want to learn more.

The good news

Imposter syndrome is:

- Not a problem

- Not an illness
- Not only you

Research shows that often high-achievers experience imposter syndrome the most. According to a review in 2020, 9%-82% of people experience imposter syndrome—everyone experiences imposter syndrome in their way.

But the good news is, feeling like you are a fraud only happens because you care. You care enough to share what you know the best way you know-how. You care because you want to serve your clients in the best way possible.

The only way forward out of this imposter syndrome loop is to move forward. Take action regardless of the fear you feel. You do not need a Ph.D., a substantial social media following, or have survived a catastrophic event to share what you know. You already know something of value that will help someone else solve their problem. They cannot do it if you are unwilling to step forward and offer the help only you can provide. If you even help only one person, you are still an expert. Who knows how many others you could help in the future if you took that first step.

Use any credentials and rave reviews you receive to market yourself and what you have to offer. You are in a different stage of life, and share your message your way. There is only one of you. Only you can express yourself most authentically. You can't improve what you offer if you aren't willing to take that first step. It would help if you were willing to take on constructive feedback and strive to do even better the next time. Progress, not perfection, is the mantra I use when my imposter syndrome rears its head. You can't be perfect and know everything. You can only try. So, put yourself out there and take one step after the other to reach your dream.

Now the bad news

The people that come to your classes don't care about you. I know that sounds harsh, but the reality is they care about what they can learn from you. They come because they are trying to solve their problems and think you can help. Your message could give them hope and the solution they have been looking for. The more you put yourself out there and help people. The more impact you can have on their lives.

Try gratitude instead

Banish imposter syndrome with thanks. Make a note of what people thank you for. As soon as people thank you for what you shared with them, you succeed. Don't be afraid to share what you know. It is the only way to tell if you are on the right track. How awesome would it be if you could change someone's life? If you don't share your genius, you can't help anyone. You also can't get validation for what you have to give. So get out there and share what you know from your heart.

CHAPTER 3 UNDERSTAND YOUR CLIENTS

Understanding your clients & how they learn

Adults learn differently than children. Adults learn best when they see practical value and relevance in learning. Teaching the exercises you choose relevant to the person you teach helps you become an engaging teacher. Adults who seek out new learning do so because they want to use the knowledge you give them. Learning is a means to an end, not an end in itself.

Often adults seek out new learning to cope with specific life-changing events. For example, marriage, divorce, a new job, a promotion, job loss, retiring, losing a loved one, moving to a new city.

In many cases, a change in circumstances prompts adults to seek new knowledge. New information helps maintain their sense of self-esteem. A solid secondary motivator is learning for pleasure.

Adults are motivated by their individual needs. Your client may not be aware that they have poor movement habits.

It is your job to guide them to understand and recognize the need for new learning. Without awareness, your clients will lack interest, attention, and motivation to learn.

Barriers to learning

Adults have responsibilities they balance against participating in an exercise class. These responsibilities create barriers to attending classes and learning new movement skills.

Some barriers include lack of:

- time
- money
- confidence
- information about the benefits of attending class
- scheduling problems
- childcare
- transport

- It is essential to consider what barriers adults face in your area and try and address them. You may want to link to a bus timetable and explain where the nearest bus stop is. You may want to have some toys available for children. Explain the benefits of your movement style in your flyers, on your website, and when talking to prospective clients.

Your potential clients are more interested in how they will benefit from coming to you. What results will they see, feel, experience by coming to class? If you can show them the relationship between attending class regularly and a tangible outcome, they will be more likely to sign up.

Understanding your clients - Adults, Teenagers, Children

Adults

Adults are people with years of experience. So, please focus on the strengths clients bring to the class, not the gaps in their knowledge. Encourage dialogue as to what clients bring to the class. Your clients' input can be a significant source of enrichment for you and them. You do not need to have all the answers; clients can be resources to you and each other.

Auditory, visual, tactile, and participatory teaching methods are all strategies you can use. Adults relate new knowledge to what they have learned before—present single concepts to your class. Make your examples relevant to practical everyday situations. For example, explain why doing thoracic extension is good to keep the spine healthy. Explain how extension exercises reverse all the sitting we do - sitting in meetings, in the car, and on the couch. Giving adults an excellent reason to change motivates them.

Be very careful not to belittle a clients' exploration of a new skill. Doing so will turn the client away from attending additional classes. Adults have pride and need support as individuals. They need to feel safe in the class. Otherwise, their self-esteem and ego are at risk.

Allow clients to admit their feelings of confusion, ignorance, or frustration. Treat all questions and comments with respect. Avoid saying 'I covered that' when someone asks a repetitive question. Adults tend to be problem-centered when learning. They generally want to apply new information or skills immediately. New skills must be relevant and meaningful to your clients. Clients can associate further details with something that they already know. If the information is similar to something a client already knows, they can revisit this learned framework or pattern.

Know what the needs are of individuals in your class. Your clients do not wish to learn what they will never use. For adult learners to be successful, there is a greater responsibility on the part of the teacher. Clients come to movement classes with defined expectations and possibly some barriers to learning. The best motivators for adult learners are interest and selfish benefit. Showing your clients how exercises benefits them, helps them perform better, and the benefits will last longer.

Children & Teenagers

Teaching children to do Pilates is fun and rewarding. Your approach needs to change from your adult classes to meet their needs. Most children have fearless personalities and a willingness to try anything. Some children will be too shy or too disinterested to take part completely. You will find yourself working to keep up with them most of the time. Children's attention spans are short, so keep class length to about 30 minutes. These classes will be wonderful and rewarding. But, there will definitely be tough days along the way.

Focus your class

You will need to be well organized to teach children's classes. Prepare a class plan and jot down some themes to build your class around. It is best to teach children mat exercises. Their bodies are too small for the apparatus. Little fingers can get caught in the springs, carriage or pedals.

Keep class numbers small and use simple language. Children won't respond to complex anatomy terms or lengthy explanations. You need to trigger their attention and find ways to keep it, or classes result in chaos. Storytelling is a great way to hook them in and introduce them to different ways to move.

Using the teaching compass model

Dorothy Heathcote developed a teacher compass that may be useful for you to consider. The compass helps you to navigate you class using an inquiry process within any given task you set.

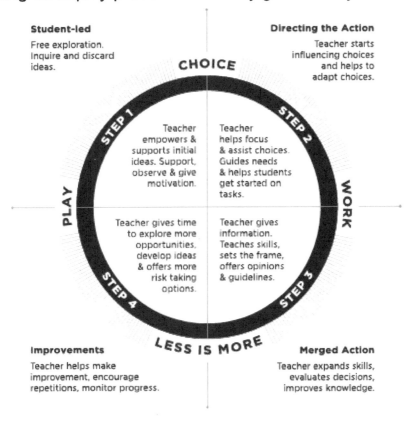

Adapted from The Circle of Progression
by Dorothy Heathcote and Gavin M. Bolton

Step 1: Student-led

Give children a task. For example, ask them to move like an animal of their choice. Identify a couple of rules for children, such as 'as we move, we are silent.' Animals like to be quiet, so they notice but don't get noticed. Mainly young children will immediately start roaring and wrestling when you ask them to be an animal. Your class will become chaotic and hard to manage otherwise.

It may also be helpful to introduce the idea of a frozen moment. Count down to a clap and then use this stillness to bring attention to a particular body aspect, such as breathing. It also helps direct the class into the next part of the lesson.

The children can explore as many animals as they like within a given time and decide which one to develop. This exploration is an excellent way for them to 'warm-up.' Encourage big actions that will use some of their boundless energy. Get them to run and explore different parts of the room, like their animal. They could touch only their elbow to a wall or nose to an object with a particular color. The teacher can make observational comments such as 'I see you are making a ...' Try not to get too involved. Stand back and see what they create.

Step 2: The teacher starts getting more involved in directing the action

The teacher provides some parameters around the action. For example, ask the children to let their animals become sleepy or run away from danger. Make sure they do this safely without hurting the other 'animals' in the room. The teacher can make additional suggestions or direct the action differently.

Step 3: The teacher now starts to merge the action.

Children could work in groups. The animals could go on a journey or prepare for a midnight party where they will dance together. Introduce some balance challenges as they walk across a 'swing bridge' as they travel. They could also carry various objects to the party and balance them on different body parts.

Step 4: Teachers sets the parameters and provides feedback

Ask the groups of children to show their story in movement. Then get the whole class to explore aspects of each group's movement vocabulary.

Storytelling

Using stories to inform movements is very powerful. You can also try using songs and include literacy and numeracy aspects. Many Pilates exercises mimic different sports or animals. You can draw on these exercises for your initial story exploration. You can also teach concepts like breathing and alignment through imagery or stories. Kids thrive on variety, so be creative and don't be afraid to try new things.

Teaching teenagers

Pilates classes for teenagers are different. Many teenagers are already participating in some high-level physical activity. They may be taking dance or gymnastics, horse riding or sport. They seek out Pilates to help them improve what they already feel competent doing. Other teenagers may have a physical ailment such as scoliosis. Teenagers may also be insecure. The physical and emotional changes they are going through are like a roller coaster.

Growth rates at this age can be unpredictable. If they have a sudden growth spurt, it is best to keep stretching very gently. Bones grow faster than muscles. End-range aggressive stretching or strengthening could do more harm than good. Incorporating some myofascial release and stretching at this stage will be more beneficial. It is gentle and does not help for long durations.

Build a positive body image & movement experience

I would also encourage you not to use mirrors in the studio as much as possible. For adolescents, the image they see in the mirror can be very confronting. They often do not see their reflection but an idea of how they look in their head. This distortion occupies their thoughts more than the exercise they are practicing.

Teaching Pilates to this age group is best done through their chosen movement activity lens. Be aware that they need a lot of positive reinforcement. As a teacher, you need to build their confidence in their changing bodies and emotions. Reassure them when these changes disrupt their physical goals. It is temporary and gives them time to focus on other aspects.

Your teenage students are taller and more muscular. Because of this, you can introduce them to Pilates equipment work. Choose exercises that nourish their passion but also assist their developing bodies. Adjust their program as their bodies change. Ask them what their goal is for the session and how you can support them. Could you give them a say and support their needs?

Teaching styles

Giving the gift of learning

Throughout our lives, we experience different teachers. Each teacher we encountered used different instructional techniques. I will assume that some of these types of teaching appealed to you more than others. These experiences may also have influenced how you go about teaching your classes.

Understanding different teaching styles and how to use them can improve how you teach Pilates.

What is meant by "teaching styles"?

The term itself has no agreed definition. But, several writers and researchers have identified particular teaching styles. They have related them to different teaching philosophies or specific learning outcomes.

There appear to be two significant findings:

1. Teaching styles have more effect when students are actively involved in the learning process.
2. Relying on personal preference is not effective in itself. So, when selecting a teaching style, do so from the knowledge point.

Each teacher's personality and individual styles of instruction are linked. Teachers make decisions about their class before a lesson. When designing a class, teachers may consider the subject matter, learning objectives, organization, and presentation.

During class time, teachers make various decisions relating to performance and execution. At the end of the lesson, the teacher considers the evaluation of performance and feedback from students to teacher and hopefully self-evaluation. The degree of responsibility the teacher or the student assumes changes throughout a lesson. When applying teaching styles to a class, there is a range of styles to choose from. Teachers may choose the direct, teacher-led approach or an open-ended, student-centered style where the teacher acts in a facilitator's role.

There is no right or wrong style of teaching. By using different styles, the teacher can meet diverse objectives within a class. The teacher might discover that the class responds better to different or multiple teaching styles by exploring other techniques. Younger children may respond better to one kind, while teenagers respond better to a different type and adult students react to yet another style.

I discuss three styles most often used. It is common for teachers to use the Command style with all age groups. This style helps to set the framework for a lesson. It helps learners become familiar with the lesson content. Then the teacher may use the Practice style to start shifting the responsibility to the learner. Teachers will still give parameters to work within. The aim is to increase their competence.

The Inclusion style allows learners to work at their level while being supported by the teacher. This style is also practical when working in an unfamiliar setting where a teacher needs to know the learners and their abilities. This style can give the teacher valuable information to structure appropriate classes for each age group or individual. Below we will explore how these styles relate to teaching movement.

Three different teaching styles

1. Command style

What it is: The teacher is responsible for making the decisions about the class. They may consider focus, location, postural imbalanced, injury history, pace and rhythm, exercise progressions, skill level, feedback, etc. The learner makes the minimum number of decisions. The learner›s role is to reproduce a precision performance that follows the teacher›s demonstration, cues, pace, and rhythm for practising movements or sequences.

Goal: Is for learners to reproduce and learn to perform the content precisely in a short period. Learners need to complete the specific objective(s).

Learning Objectives: Students will be able to accurately reproduce movements shown in class. Learners are given a predetermined model and expected to demonstrate skill acquisition. This style of teaching allows the teacher to cover more material.

Behavioral Objectives: The learners achieve conformity and uniformity. Learners can follow directions on cue, adhere to a particular discipline, and perform specific standards.

2. Practice style

What it is: This teaching style is part of the developmental process of independence. It progresses learning on from the initial command style of learning. The teacher makes all subject matter and logistical decisions and provides private feedback to the learners. The role of the learner is to individually and privately practice a task while completing a variety of decisions. These decisions may include where they will practice, what to wear, the order of the movements or exercises, the starting time, pace and rhythm they will use, when they will rest and when to stop practising. Learners can reflect in their own time and may plan questions. They can seek clarification at a later time with their teacher's guidance.

Objectives: The learner will be able to practice by themself and correctly reproduce the movements. The learner can recall cognitive memories and perform the exercise (s). They use repetition to internalize the actions. It stimulates their internal feedback.

Behavioral objectives: Learners gain independence. They make decisions and develop the ability to initiate skill acquisition. This ability to make their own decisions helps them to be accountable for the consequence of each decision, for example:

- the relationship between the effort involved and the time it takes to achieve the result they want
- pacing each session to avoid over-training or practising a movement with incorrect alignment and possibly sustaining an injury.

They learn to develop trust in their abilities to make good decisions.

3. Inclusion style

What it is: The defining characteristic of the Inclusion style is that people with varying degrees of skill can participate in the same class. Design the class with multiple degrees of difficulty in mind. Learners can select a level of difficulty to practice a movement. They have the choice of the level they are going to attempt first. If necessary, they can then make some decisions to adjust their choice. They also have the option of making self-assessment decisions. In some cases, guidelines set by the teacher helps to inform their decisions.

The teachers' role is to make all subject matter decisions. Teachers also set the different levels in the task. The teacher then steps back and observes learners as they explore deciding where to start interacting with the task. The teacher can step in from time to time to offer support as a coach, facilitator, motivator, or advisor. Teachers need to draw on their observation skills. They must listen and provide appropriate input to help learners develop their initiative.

The role of the learner is to consider the available levels in the task. They select a starting point and practice the task. They are responsible for making adjustments in the task level and checking their performance against the criteria.

Objectives: The teacher can accommodate individual performance differences by designing a range of options for students to explore a new movement sequence/movement idea. Students use different tools to develop new movement content. The teacher provides opportunities for continued participation. Learners will be able to make ongoing decisions and develop self-assessment skills.

Behavioral objectives: Learners make decisions about approaching a task by choosing an initial level of performance for themselves. They can then practice self-evaluation skills using a performance criterion and make adjustment decisions to continue participating.

Learners may accept the reality of their differences in physical and performance abilities. They will learn to deal with similarities or discrepancies between their aspiration and the reality of their performance. Developing these objectives can help students gain a sense of self-reliance and honesty in self-evaluation.

Example

Initially, you may teach a class using the Command style to discuss and demonstrate the importance of a particular movement or sequence and model the correct way of performing the activity.

You can then use the Practice style and invite participants to reflect on your demonstration by asking questions rather than giving answers. For example, "What are some essential things you must remember when …? A variety of solutions will make discussion possible and allow you to check their understanding. Follow this with an opportunity for everyone to practice the movement several times with your guidance.

If working with a larger group of older children or teenagers, you can divide the participants into groups and ask them to work together to refine the movement(s). Younger children will respond better to a rich imaginary world. It is a creative way to use the command style but allows the younger children to participate while teaching them specific techniques in a fun way.

When working with teens, you might ask students to come back to their next lesson with their movement or movement sequence that incorporates the task learned in class. They can share their movement sequence with the other students. The teacher will then be able to use their movement ideas to facilitate learning through the Inclusion style.

Encourage adults to practice the movement(s) at least twice more at home. If they need equipment and don't have any available, they could use visualization to imagine doing the movements. It also helps to link practice to an everyday task. For example, do a balance exercise while washing dishes or brushing teeth. They can use the time they are already using for a repetitive task. No extra time is needed to practice.

It is beneficial for a teacher to use various teaching styles to encourage broad learner engagement and learning. Different people are attracted to different styles, so you are broadening your capacity to reach and motivate them.

Feedback

Two types of feedback

There are two significant types of feedback -- intrinsic and extrinsic. The feedback you provide gives clients information to change their movement habits.

Giving clients corrections every time they move leads them to rely less on themselves. They become over-reliant on you. Think of this two-way discovery process as a way to foster independence. Give your clients options and wait for them to respond. You can also ask them questions or encourage them to do the movement differently.

One of the difficulties experienced by many clients is that they frequently get too much feedback, leading to an overload of information. Establishing an understanding of baseline biomechanical actions and allowing time for them to practice the movements will make giving feedback easier.

Intrinsic feedback

Intrinsic feedback is the sensory information that usually occurs when you move. This information is derived from sources outside the body (visual or auditory) or inside the body (proprioception).

Benefits: It gives the body indications such as the positions of the joints or orientation within space. Intrinsic feedback is always present and can assist clients in determining when they are doing something incorrectly. It can also help a client to recognise improvements when executing exercises.

Drawbacks: Intrinsic signals will not always clarify the precise reason why a movement was successful or unsuccessful or how to improve the movement execution in the future

Extrinsic feedback

The teacher plays a vital role by providing extrinsic feedback. It is beneficial to focus on the correct form and where immediate feedback for safety is needed or expected by the learner.

Drawbacks: Avoid providing corrections every time a client moves. The client can become reliant on external error correction and less on themselves. A heavy focus on error correction may cause the client to 'switch off' their intrinsic signals. They rely solely on extrinsic feedback.

Benefits: Regardless of the type of feedback used, one of the most important functions is to provide motivation. Motivation and goal achievement are linked. When a client feels they are making progress, their motivation levels increase. Positive feedback will reinforce a client's motivation and confidence. It makes it more likely that they will repeat actions successfully again.

Giving praise

When complimenting a client, praise the specific action. Being clear promotes learning. Acknowledge improvements overtime to support changes in a client's movements.

Develop your communication style

Teaching a class with multiple participants requires you to monitor a group and make specific corrections. You will also need to motivate clients of different abilities within the class.

Your biggest challenge will be keeping the group focussed while assisting one client. It takes time and experience to develop this skill. But, it all starts with the first step.

How is communication like a pancake?

Making pancakes and teaching movements have a lot in common. Leadership and education training often use this theory to teach communication strategies. It is a valuable communication framework for teaching movement too. Think of how you felt about teaching your first class. You may have experienced it as challenging and a little patchy. You may also have over analysed your approach, had a lot of self-doubts and were way too hard on yourself. But, you lived to see another day.

First attempts are often like a first pancake - a little misshaped and lumpy. Your students probably didn't even notice your rough start and crippling self-doubt. The same goes for movements our clients do. Observe the first couple of repetitions before giving feedback. The body needs time to become familiar with a move. The first movement is often crusty and irregular - like the first pancake. It gets better as they go along and can be even more exciting with your guidance. Allow your client to get familiar with the movement before adding your feedback into the mix.

There are three key communication lessons we can learn from pancakes.

1. You can't see the other side of the pancake by only looking at the top side.

   You don't know what the other person is thinking about a topic until you share and discuss it with them. Then their side of the pancake becomes a little clearer.

2. You have to flip the pancake to see the other side.

To understand the other person's point of view, you have to invest some effort. To see the other side of the pancake by turning it over. It takes effort. To understand how someone sees the world, you have to make an effort. Ask questions, be curious. Give them a chance to explain their point of view.

3. The centre of the pancake is more tender than the outside edges.

Our view of what the other person thinks is a little crusty on the outside. We need to break through to the middle to get to the heart of any matter. The centre of the pancake is more sensitive. We should listen without judging and then seek clarification.

Taking this approach also helps us to be curious. We can be more aware of what clients think, feel, and experience. To gain more clarity, ask some questions. Questions help you to check-in. You can assess if the way you used language to describe something resonated with them. Do they understand your word choices in the way you meant it?

What motivates your clients?

Motivation walks hand in hand with goal achievement. Making progress towards your goals increases your motivation. As a movement teacher, you are helping clients to reach their goals. We do this by assisting them to gain intrinsic feedback and encouragement. Intrinsic motivators foster belief in the value of looking after your body and movement health. Developing an awareness of our sensory system will build our perception more.

Intrinsic motivation tools can also help you to foster committed clients. Focus on making the exercises you teach relevant to each client. For example, incorporate clients' personal experiences into lessons. You can also discuss the reasons for choosing specific exercises. You can figure out how certain tasks fit your client's everyday life. Making connections to previous learning can also help. We all learn by doing, making, writing, designing, creating or problem-solving. Telling clients what to do makes them passive, and they expect you to provide all the answers. It reduces their curiosity.

Instead, encourage clients to suggest approaches to problems and become active class participants. Then allow them to practice the movements. Invite them to explore and verbalise what they feel.

Learning Styles

Understanding how your clients learn helps you meet their educational needs fundamentally. Each person's reality is unique. How you perceive an event is different to someone else. Everyone sees, hears, feels and experiences life in their way. We all have a specific way of learning. We may use a combination of styles when learning a new skill.

Some experiences lend themselves better to certain styles of learning. For example, experiencing a piece of music will be mostly auditory (A). But, some people may also see images (V) while others feel the 'mood' of the piece (K). Others may be more internally focused and running a commentary (Ad) about the experience.

People operate in all of these symbolic systems but tend to process or rely mainly on one of these systems. People's behaviour within their dominant style is pretty typical. We can categorise the styles as:

Visual (V): You create and see pictures in your mind. A visual style allows you to assimilate and compare a large amount of information and compare it to what you already know. Visual learners talk fast. They find verbal instructions harder to recall. They need to see something to make sense and are easily distracted by noise.

Mainly visual people operate more from the top half of their bodies. They tend to breathe shallowly and speak faster. They stand or sit with their bodies erect and look upward. They sit at the front of the chair. Appearances are important to them. They tend to be more organised and neat and are often wiry in their build. They learn by associating images with ideas. Verbal instructions are more challenging for them to recall. They aren't easily distracted by noise, and they need to see something to capture their attention and interest.

Auditory (A): This learning style is more sequential, and you take longer to process information. It lends contrast to visual learning, like the soundtrack to a movie. They are easily distracted by noise and feel loved by your choice of words and tone of voice. People who are mainly auditory breathe from the middle of their chests. They move their eyes from side to side, often talk to themselves and are distracted by noise. They learn by hearing information sequentially. Tell auditory learners how they are doing. These learners feel understood by certain tones of voice or words. They like talking on the phone and listening to music.

Kinaesthetic (K): These learners use sensory experiences without evaluation. They explore the world through their internal proprioceptive system and external tactile sensation experience. They respond to touch and physical rewards like hugs. They learn and memorise by doing. The movement has to feel right. They typically breathe from the bottom of their lungs. Their stomach will visibly move, and they speak slowly. They respond to touch and physical rewards. They learn by doing. Something has to 'feel right' for them to become interested.

Auditory-digital (self-talk/AD): This style is related to what people say to themselves. Their internal self-talk about events and experiences. They make decisions based on a list of criteria. They use any or all of the representative systems and respond to things' making sense'. They often listen to inner dialogue in their heads. They make decisions based on a list of criteria and are interested in something 'making sense'. They use any or all of the other learning styles too.

Learning Style Test

We all use one learning style over another. This is your preferred or primary representational system or learning style.

A.

Take the test

Do the learning styles test and then score your answers in the boxes below.

For each of the following statements place a number next to each phrase.

4=Almost always

3=Often

2=Sometimes

1=Almost never

1. I make a choice when

____It feels right to me

____I hear it, and it sounds right to me

____I see it, and it looks right to me

____I review it, and it fits my criteria

- When discussing and issue, I am persuaded by:

____How convincing the person sounds

____Seeing the other's point of view

____How reasonable the individual makes the point

____My gut feeling

- When I meet someone for the first time, I am impressed by:

____The appearance of the person

____How he or she makes me feel

____How articulate or intelligent the individual is

____If what the person says rings true to me

- I generally respond to:

____Sounds, I am easily distracted by noises

____Interesting facts, distracted by my thoughts

____Sensations, distracted by how my own body feels

____Sights, distracted by colours around me

- 5 When I like a proposal, I tend to say things like:

____Sounds good

____Makes sense

____Got it!

____Looks good

B. Copy the number values from your test in the same sequence you wrote them

1	2	3	4.	5
K	A	V	A	A
A	V	K	Ad	Ad
V	Ad	Ad	K	K
Ad	K	A	V	V

C. Record each number in the corresponding box and then add each column

Question	Visual	Auditory	Kinesthetic	Auditory - digital
1				
2				
3				
4				
5				

Total				

The scores in each column will give the relative preference for each of the four primary learning styles. The highest total will be your preferred learning style

CHAPTER 4 TOOLKIT

Pilates teaching tools

Demonstration

The purpose of showing an exercise is to increase your client's understanding of Pilates. You do so by providing an accurate 'picture' or model of the movement. But the client may, in some cases, not perform the exercise accurately. Then other tools such as explanation and questioning assist in clarifying the activity.

Curiosity stimulates problem-solving and gives the motivation to learn a new skill. You can also use more tools. For example, break down a complex exercise into parts. You teach each piece and allow the client to slow down and improve the movement. Verbal cues help to clarify the actions.

When observing a client doing an exercise, do so from various angles. Then ask questions to check their understanding. There are multiple opportunities within each session to show clients an exercise.

1. when introducing a new exercise
2. as a reminder, in the next exercise class
3. at the end of an exercise as a final reminder

Explanation complements demonstration. But it is essential first to show the exercise without verbal cues. Demonstration without talking helps the client focus on the movement pattern without distraction. After that, give them one verbal cue to focus on when starting the exercise.

Explanation

The explanation of an exercise is a component of demonstration. A description is an opportunity for the teacher to talk and the client to listen. This instructional strategy introduces, provides or expands information given to the client.

It is necessary to gain and maintain a client's full attention. Keep the explanation brief and state the main focus for the exercise. These explanations need to lead to physical practice so the client can learn.

Create a routine of planning an instruction sequence

This discipline will increase the exercise time in a class. Consider the following points when planning an exercise session:

1. Are you planning to introduce a new skill(s)?
2. How will you introduce it?
3. What language will help the client identify with the movement?
4. How and when will you use demonstration/explanation?
5. Which aspect of the exercise do you want the client to focus on?
6. What are the critical points for each exercise?

Guidelines for explanation techniques

When explaining a new concept to clients, try to:

1. Avoid explaining during demonstrations
2. Demonstrations and explanations must complement each other.
3. Keep your explanations brief
4. Focus on explaining one issue at a time
5. Provide an opportunity for physical practice before moving onto a new issue
6. Assist client's understanding through the use of imagery, touch and cue words
7. Question clients to determine their understanding of the explanations

Questioning

Asking meaningful questions will increase learning. When clients are encouraged to think for themselves and understand their bodies responses to exercise, they will achieve better results. Questioning generates a problem-solving mode of thinking with clients, and it will assist them in taking ownership of the solutions they formulate.

Questioning needs to adapt to each situation because the questions stimulate discovery and creativity.

The right time to ask a question is an art, and unfortunately, there is no formula. Gaining a client's attention at the right moment helps. It may take time for clients to become comfortable with this instructional tool, but as learning progresses, they will become more involved in their learning process as their skills increase. When clients respond to questions and offer solutions, you should encourage their ideas, no matter how vague or incomplete they perceive them. If a client finds sincere support from you, they will be more likely to respond the next time you ask a question.

If you start by establishing a safe environment where clients feel confident to voice their responses to questions, they will likely be more motivated to answer them in the future. There are two ways to formulate questions - simple or complex. Each approach has a different way of question formulation.

a. Simple Questions

When a client needs to remember specific ideas and concepts, simple questions are appropriate.

They can also serve as reminder cues. These are factual questions with only one possible answer and are generally what? or where? questions like: *What position is your pelvis in when doing the Hundred exercise?*

b. Complex Questions

Complex questions stimulate abstract thinking. They provide self-evaluation opportunities and assist clients in making informed decisions about their bodies outside their sessions. With this question style, you give them the tools to analyse, evaluate, apply, and create knowledge related to their bodies.

Formulate these questions with the client's existing level of body knowledge in mind. Give your clients time to consider their answers. It is tempting to answer on their behalf, but this will stop them from taking ownership of the 'problem'. Re-phrasing the question if needed to clarify what you are asking. Use comparison to an ideal model when formulating complex questions. Then ask What? Where? and How? questions to clarify the exercise purpose.

After that, allow the client to experience the exercise several times with the correct form. An example of a complex question is:

How will you find your neutral pelvic alignment?

Guidelines for structuring your questions

- Consider the nature of the exercise a client is trying to master
- Rehearse the questions by writing them down and saying them out loud to yourself
- Make sure you have a variety of simple and complex questions
- Plan your questions to lead automatically to a known answer but make sure you do not expect your clients to be mind-readers if there are a variety of options opened up to your questioning structure
- Formulate your questions based on your clients' existing knowledge
- If you are working with an individual for the first time, you will need to ask questions that inform you about their level of knowledge

Imagery

Your body responds to the way you think, feel and act. When you feel stressed, anxious or upset, your body may try to tell you something is not correct. It does this by increasing your blood pressure, back pain or headaches. This mind-body connection is a great tool to use when teaching movement.

Imagery can help your clients integrate thought, emotion and action when processing information. Using imagery in a movement class can assist your teaching, especially when the verbal description and physical demonstration need more clarification. Most of the studies about mental training show that it improves motor skills.

It may also enhance confidence, motivation and mental toughness. Images can help you reinforce what you want out of a movement.

For example, if you want a supple spine, you can imagine your spine moving like a panther. Your mind flashes images, thoughts, and notions approximately 50,000 times a day. Your posture, the way you move and the discomfort you feel link to these 'flashes'. We can tap into positive, constructive thoughts to create powerful, dynamic bodies. The use of language is one of our most powerful tools when teaching clients to do their exercise programmes, but frequently, there are limitations when trying to describe an action verbally. Imagery can assist in expressing ideas that are too subtle for speech.

The reason visual imagery works is because you imagine yourself performing a movement. You are creating neural patterns in your brain as if you had physically done the action. These patterns are like small tracks engraved in the brain cells. These 'tracks' enable you to move better by mentally practising the move. The intention behind using mental imagery is to train your mind. You create the neural patterns in your brain to teach your body to do what you want it to do. To do anything in life, you need a clear picture of what you want to achieve and a plan for how to fulfil it. To improve movement, you need to increase your ability to be more aware. It takes courage, consistent practice, clear intention, desire, and faith to enjoy using imagery. In the process, you will let go of physical tension. Allowing tension to dissolve can release emotions. Some clients may be too attached to the familiarity of being tense. It may be too frightening

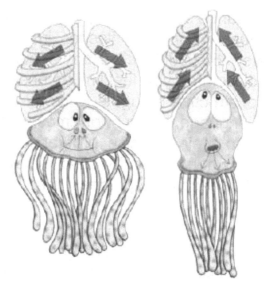

Jellyfish breathing

  Imagery can establish a sense of positive well-being. The good news is you can learn to use imagery at any stage of learning and any age. It creates the capacity to improve learning skills and performance. You may choose to take an internal or external view. Meaning that you can imagine doing the movement - internal view. If you choose to watch yourself performing the exercise, you will take an external view. You should use the 'view' that best suits your personality or the situation.

Seed Images

Seed images are starter images to help you explain concepts like posture or releasing tension from the body. You can suggest and ask your client if the image resonates or if something else comes to mind for them that is more appropriate.

Hot air balloon

Your pelvis is the basket of a hot air balloon. Your abdominals are the ropes that keep the basket and balloon apart. Your rib cage and head are the coloured silk balloon. Your breath is the flame that lifts you into the air. Your feet will resemble gravity trying to pull you back down to earth.

Melt tension away

We often 'try' too hard when we want to relax an area of the body. Try asking a client to melt their shoulders and see what happens. Better yet, try doing this yourself. What image came to mind? Ice cream or chocolate melting on a hot summer day?

Touch

Clear dialogue

Touch is a dialogue between the teacher and client. You or your client always have the right to decline touch. It would help if you were clear on your intent when using touch. Hesitant touch may cause discomfort to your client. It will also interfere with the learning process. Your touch needs to be gentle but firm. Pain in response to touch is rarely suitable as it causes the muscles to contract and protect. Pain can be helpful when it makes the teacher and the client aware of sensitivity in the body. Planning touch is complex, and it relies a lot on your intuition. You will develop your touch techniques over time. Being open to messages from clients will help in developing appropriate touch techniques. Ask clients for feedback from time to time. Check that your touch technique and their experience of your touch is proper. Your client is the expert. They know a lot more about how they experience touch.

Consent cards: You can use a consent card in group classes. The cards allow the client to indicate if touch correction is acceptable or not in a group situation. The card has the word yes on one side and no on the other. Using cards means clients who do not want to receive touch do not have to speak up in class. They place the card next to their space with the correct word facing up. The teacher can then provide the appropriate guidance as they move around the room.

Touch cue formula

Touch cues require concentration from both people. When applying touch, you first move your focus to your hands. Then move your focus to the area of the client's body you are touching. This slight pause gives the client time to focus on the site you are handling. You can also encourage clients to apply self-touch. You can also cue **self-touch** to help clients understand what you mean and build intrinsic feedback. This is also useful when you are not able to use touch correction like when you are teaching online.

General guidelines for a confident touch

a. Palm or flat finger pressure: Firm, direct pressure through these parts of the hand covers a large body area. It is secure and comforting. It minimises tickling. Tickling causes the muscle to contract and register confusion in the nerve endings.

b. Brushing: Stimulate surface proprioception with this type of touch. It brings general awareness to an area. Your client will feel this touch as either a pleasant stroking sensation or a subtle friction sensation.

c. Directional: With your palm flat on a body part, encourage movement in the direction you want the limb or joint to move. Directional touch is useful for subtle, small movements within joints.

d. Massage balls: You can add another dimension to your touch by using tools like spiky balls or massage rollers. They allow indirect contact. These tools may be more comfortable for the client until you can establish a level of trust.

Cueing styles

Effective cueing can differentiate between an excellent movement session and a not so great one. Many exercises are complex. When you communicate how to move, you use both demonstration and words.

Your words matter: The words you use will significantly affect the outcome of an exercise. Keep your word choices simple. Complex words can cause confusion rather than understanding. Choose words that convey the quality of movement you want. Try this when cueing a basic abdominal curl. 'Float your head' rather than 'lift your head'. It can make a difference to how people experience an abdominal strengthening exercise.

Your client's quality of movement can change once you start changing your words. The words and range of techniques you draw on will help your clients interpret your teaching.

Clients have different modes of learning, visual, kinaesthetic or auditory. In general, each person may draw on a combination of these modes. We are all more inclined to one in particular. Visual learners like to see the exercise demonstrated. Auditory learners want an explanation. Explanations can be analytical or figurative (use of imagery). Kinaesthetic learners respond to touch and like to do the exercises immediately.

People learn through doing and making changes as they go along. You will find that not all clients respond the same to all cues. It would help if you remained flexible when choosing your cues. Be willing to change your instructions if they confuse a client. Creative cueing is a continuous journey of discovery, and your inspiration can come from many sources. Sources may include books, online videos, or taking a class taught by other teachers.

Make new cues your own

Sometimes 'borrowing' cues from other instructors can be clunky. You may be uncomfortable with the cues you are using. Your clients will pick up on your discomfort. So, when you use a borrowed concept, find your way of describing the material. Practice it out loud on your own. Try and record yourself and play the recording back. Listen to your explanation and tweak it for more clarity.

When teaching this new cue, watch your class to determine if your choice of words works. If people have confused looks, it might be time to reconsider your words. Find another way to articulate the quality of movement you want. Be aware that sexual humour cues may be funny for some and offensive to others. It is best to steer clear of this type of cue at all times.

Over time you will become more able to combine various cueing techniques. You will also become more adept at using multiple cueing and teaching tools for a situation. Successful cueing strategies involves many layers, such as learning, practising, experiencing, observing, evaluating and tapping into one's intuition.

Five steps for cueing success

1. Learn, practice and understand the exercise on every level. It would help increase your anatomical, biomechanical, and teaching method understanding.
2. Film yourself teaching. Then become your client. Listen to your cues. Do they make sense? Does your class flow? What is the speed of your cue delivery? It may surprise you to learn that you need to talk faster than the movement occurs. Your client needs to hear what to do next a fraction before doing it. When evaluating your recording be kind to yourself. Remember, this is a journey of discovery. Don't beat yourself up for your mistakes. Learn from them and work on improving the way you teach. It is fun.
3. Practice using a variety of cueing techniques. Observe how they translate to movement on different bodies.
4. Focus on your clients. Become familiar with the client's skill level, capability, restrictions, and injuries. Keep these in mind when designing and delivering your classes.
5. Set goals and objectives for yourself to teach the exercises or class. It is possible to find motivation for yourself while keeping your clients needs in mind.

Choosing the best type of cue speeds progress and creates positive movement experiences. There are a variety of cue types you can draw on to help clients move well:

Cue types

1. Anatomical/form cues

Use anatomical cues that align with your clients' level of knowledge. Few clients know where *Serratus Anterior* or *Gluteus Medius* is. But most people can relate to their ribs, shoulder blades or front of the thigh.

As a teacher, you can increase your client›s knowledge. Show them pictures or use a skeleton to explain where specific key/bones muscles sit in the body. These mini-educational sessions are not for everyone. For those that want to move, use cues like «*feel length between the crown of the head and the tailbone*", "*soften your breastbone*", or "*push off from your big toe*". These cues will give your client enough information about which part of their body to move.

2. Imagery cues:

These cues are fun and creative. This type of cue is effective for visual learners. Our brains interpret images more than words. The wrong image can interrupt this effectiveness. Images can create confusion. If this is the case, ask clients if they understand how the image relates to the movement. If so, ask them to give you an idea they associate with the action.

3. Sound cues

Sound cues are great to distract clients when they hold their breath or for auditory learners. They associate the sound with the movement. I had a client once that I could direct through sound cues. Even in a group class, I could make a particular sound, and this client would adjust their body. I didn't have to say anything else. A sound cue can be like yelling SURPRISE randomly. It makes people pay attention. Sound cues are also great when clients carry a lot of tension in their necks and jaws. Use a long slow 'ahhhhh' sound for a basic abdominal curl. Clients may feel a bit self-conscious at first. But, adding some sound encourages breathing and a softer jaw and neck. You can also ask clients to hum on an exhale or sing. Sounds may also help clients who try too hard. It allows them to relax into a movement. They have something else to think about as they perform an exercise.

4. Directional cues

Many clients struggle to differentiate between left and right when they are exercising. It makes it much easier when you use landmarks in the room you are teaching to orient your client. For example, ask your client to rotate their torso towards the door or away from the stereo. They could lengthen a leg towards the ceiling or reach their fingers towards their heels.

5. Descriptive cues

Words like squeeze, push or pull will often interrupt a movement. The client is more likely to do a quick, gripped muscle activation. For example, *squeezing your glute muscles* may lead to the pelvis tucking, resulting in losing alignment. Try cueing the client to draw the sitting bones toward each other. Or to move the muscles from the outside of the hip around toward the sitting bones. Clients can find improvement in their movement patterns.

6. Tactile cues

Some clients prefer touch to assist their understanding. Physical contact can be direct and time-efficient. Ask your client permission to use touch. In a group class, you can use consent cards. Clients can then choose if they would like to receive touch correction or not. If you are comfortable receiving touch, you can also allow the client to touch you. This sensation can help them when they are doing the exercise. You can also cue clients to self-touch. When using touch, be professional, deliberate and confident. If you or the client is uncomfortable with touch, choose other cueing methods. Using physical contact has many possible implications and misinterpretations. Take care when using this type of cue.

Anatomy of a cue

Creating effective cues is both an art and a science. It takes a lot of practice and tweaking until you find what works for you. No two people teach the same way. Only you can teach the way you do. Below is one approach to creating a formula for your cues. There will always be exceptions to this rule, but it is good to start. This formula will help you become more comfortable with layering your cues. If clients start getting distracted with the breath cue, switch the procedure. Describe the movement first, then allow them to practice before you ask them to add the breath cue. It takes time and practice. Reassure them that it is not a problem. Practice helps. Mental stress in response to movement is counterproductive. Make sure they move first always. Add the breath after they get comfortable with the movement.

1. Know the exercise you are going to teach

It is tough to be creative and precise when trying to teach something you don't know how to do. Practice the exercises and understand them in your own body. Teach what you love first. It will help build your confidence.

2. Cue the position

Start by cueing the client into the position you want them to be in. For example, *Lie on your back. Knees bent—heels in line with your sitting bones*. Or, *lie on your side facing the windows. Lengthen your legs away from the crown of your head. Stack your hips over each other...*

3. Breath or movement?

Next, you need to choose if you will start the exercise by leading with the breathing or the movement. If the action is a little complicated, I tend to start teaching the movement and then adding the breath. But it is up to you and your client which order you use step 3. Play with it and see what works best for you.

4. Layer your cues

When your client grasps the movement and can combine it with breathing, you can start adding other cues. Please give them a cue and wait for them to repeat it once or twice before adding another. It would help if you gave clients time to try and put your words into practice before giving them something else to add. You don't need to share everything you know in one session. It takes time for a body to learn new ways to move. Stay calm and be patient.

5. Stay calm

It takes time and mental focus to improve the way you cue. If something doesn't work, try another approach. Your client is unlikely to know what you were trying to do didn't work. Stay calm. Stop. Think. Breathe. It will be better next time.

6. Ask for help

If you are struggling, ask for help from a more experienced teacher.

Using storytelling when teaching movement

Telling a good story is a powerful way to motivate people to reach their goals. Stories can also help you make a Pilates class fun and memorable. Storytelling helps you engage your client's emotions and give them essential information. But telling stories requires insight and skill. You need to present the information to your client in a memorable way.

The role of problem-solving in learning

Filmmaker Andrew Stanton states:

> "Make the audience put things together. Don't give them 4. Give them 2+2. The elements you provide. The order you place them in is crucial to whether you succeed or fail at engaging the audience. The audience wants to work for their meal. They don't want to know they are doing that."

Adults tend to have a problem-centred approach to learning. They generally want to apply new information or skills to current situations immediately. So new knowledge and skills must be relevant to the concerns of clients. Your clients don't want to learn what they'll never use.

You've had stories instilled in you since you were a child. You've read books, watched great movies, attended the theatre. A well-told story makes you a promise that it will lead somewhere that is worth your time. A well-told promise propels you through the story to the end. Stories are also instrumental in how we remember. We assemble bits and pieces of experience into narratives. Storytelling has no fast rules. But here are some of some elements that make a story compelling.

A 'good' story should:

- have a central theme
- invoke a sense of wonder as it develops
- draw on your personal experiences
- express values that resonate deep down inside you
- provide elements that help you problem-solve.

When is storytelling useful in a movement class?

A good story can:

1. prompt your client's memory
2. help them create movement quality and flow
3. help you structure your class.

A list of movements used to describe an exercise from beginning to end is bland & unmemorable. Complex exercises challenge our memory while changing shape and transitioning from one position to another. It can be tricky to keep track of these changes.

If you have ever tried to remember a list of random words, you'll know it is hard to do. But, if you weave the words into a story, you have a better chance of remembering them. In the same way, a good story can aid your client's memory. A story can also create the movement quality and flow you want to see, and your clients want to feel, in their bodies.

How to uncover a story

1. Ask questions

Start by finding out what your client needs to do to restore balance to their body. Identifying a purpose for exercises can help inspire a good body story.

Then consider what keeps your client (or group of clients) from achieving their goal. Ask questions that will help you understand your client's way of thinking.

What images come to mind for them when they do a particular movement?

2. Planning

Now consider the parts of the story.

Setting — where does the story take place?

The setting includes the place and the atmosphere, time, and situation. The more detailed, the better. Imagine the location for your story:

- The place — a city, forest, or beach.
- The surrounding — such as the type of building. What is the colour of the walls? What furniture is in it?
- Smells, the season, the weather

Characters — who is the story about?

These can be real people, animals, or made-up creatures like monsters, fairies, or angels. Consider the following elements with example suggestions.

- Personality — excitement, an air of anticipation.
- Physical characteristics — everyone is smiling and laughing. They are sad, energetic or angry.
- The characters' past. Could there be a backstory with other characters?
- Their conflicts — worried, disappointed, others may be happy and full of energy.
- The problems they face — social interactions such as being shy uncomfortable. Others may be comfortable, confident, happy.
- What motivates them? Do they want to take part in the action but feel scared?

Plot – what happens in the story?

Let's imagine we are going to a party. Can you identify the Pilates exercise from the story?

Introduction — characters, setting, and the event that gives rise to the conflict

- Arriving at the party.
- Putting weights on your shoulders.
- Tying helium balloons on your wrists that float your arms up.

Rising action — the furthering of that conflict

- Having to greet someone by shaking their hand across a large table.
- Take care to bend over the birthday cake without crushing it.

Conflict — a struggle between two forces

Multi-tasking: draw your belly away from the birthday cake. AND reach forward to shake someone's hand.

Climax – the turning point of the story. It's the most intense part!

- When you have to do the exercise again.
- Or if you spot a client who is crushing the cake!

Theme — the central insight of the story

Keep your shoulders relaxed. Engage your abdominals when you lean forward, and for goodness sake, don't ruin the birthday cake!

If you guessed the exercise *Saw*, you are correct!

3. Try it yourself

Try using a combination of these elements and plan a story of your own.

CHAPTER 5 ENVIRONMENTS

Teaching environments

Teaching in person

When teaching movement classes, you find different posture types, fitness, and health levels. Take time to talk to your clients at the beginning of each class. You can use this time to assess their ability to participate. Keep their limitations in mind as you progress through your class and modify exercises accordingly. You will also need to keep in mind the timing of the session and the level of the client(s).

Using the primary spinal movements of flexion, extension, side flexion, and rotation, you can create specific exercise frameworks that help clients as they improve their postural alignment, strength and flexibility. If a client experiences pain or considerable discomfort, ask them to stop. They can:

- assume a rest position like child's pose or
- lie on their back, hugging their knees to their chest.

You may need to modify the exercise to accommodate a specific client's problem. For example, a client with osteoporosis should not do flexion work. Keep their heads on the ground during abdominal strengthening exercises and focus on breathing and stable alignment when working on strengthening exercises.

You can also give clients a few alternatives before starting an exercise.

Example: rolling up the mats to sit on to help gain a comfortable sitting position when hamstrings are too short. Or, if they have wrist issues, they could do some exercises on their forearms or place their hands on a rolled-up mat instead of palms flat on the ground.

Staying safe

You can help prevent problems and potential injuries by being safety conscious. The safety of all people in the studio is always essential, and instructors have a special responsibility to be extra vigilant and anticipate any problems. By thinking about how your actions can help avoid unnecessary risks or potential injuries, you can help prevent hazards from developing into problems.

Only allow bottled water with secure leak-free tops in the studio and ask your clients to place them out of the way.

Encourage clients to remove jewellery before coming into the room. If they remove their glasses, place them in a safe place where they cannot be damaged or cause injury to another participant or the teacher.

Mat classes

When working with groups, set up the mat class space yourself. Place the mats and other equipment you want to use in a way that is easy to reach but makes it possible to move around the room without tripping. Place the equipment at the 'head end' of the mat helps to not get in the way. As you arrange the room, you can do a safety check on all pieces of equipment as you lay them out.

Equipment space

A bi-weekly check of all equipment will help maintain quality and safety standards. **Regular maintenance helps keep all the equipment in top working condition. If anyth**ing breaks or becomes damaged, it could interrupt our ability to use the studio.

Below are a few guidelines to keep in mind when using the equipment.

- Always do a safety check before starting to work on any machine
- Remind your client that their hands and body should be free of oil or sweat. The presence of either could lead to them slipping or losing their grip
- Always replace used equipment immediately so the studio area remains free of clutter
- Always clean the equipment surfaces after use. I recommend a weak solution of 10 drops of tea tree oil or eucalyptus oil in a litre of water.

Spray and wipe the surfaces with a soft, lint free cloth.

- Should anything break, stop using the equipment piece immediately
- Encourage clients to bring water bottles with secure, leak-free tops. Never place water on or near the equipment
- Set all springs before anyone gets on to the machine
- Ask clients to sit up and wait a few seconds before getting off the equipment

When a misunderstanding occurs

Clients have made a significant decision to come for Pilates classes. They may also have high expectations of the effectiveness of Pilates. So, in your dealings with them by phone and in person, your focus should be on being responsive, polite and fair.

Very rarely, there will be a misunderstanding or a mistake. What matters is that you resolve such issues in a patient and helpful way. Don't try to investigate who made a mistake.

You should always apologise for the confusion. Even when it looks like the client has got mixed up, make every effort to sort it out to their satisfaction. It is much easier to lose a client than to gain a new one. Once a client is unhappy, they are likely to tell others, including many potential new clients.

Your clients first class

The most sensitive time for a studio workout client is their first class. It is easy to forget that the client will be nervous. Their first response to the apparatus is that they look threatening and strange.

Bear in mind that their experience begins at the front door.

- Introduce yourself at the door and make the client welcome. Invite them to remove their shoes and go ahead of you into the studio. This short walk provides an early sign of posture and gait for a teacher.
- Invite the client to fill out the medical history questionnaire if they did not do it online and offer them a drink of water. If they have coats and bags, suggest placing them to one side.

- While the client is filling in the form, you should be in the studio and be available to answer any questions. When they have completed the questionnaire, discuss the main points with the client. Attempt to build up a clear picture of their health and needs. Discuss their goals. You may need to make extra notes as they arise from the discussion.
- If the client needs to change, show them to the changing room.

The first class introduces your clients to the history and principles of Pilates. The class should also connect to their goals.

At the end of a class

- At the end of the class, book your client in for their next class. Record the client's appointment on your schedule for the appropriate day and time.
- Invite the client to make their payment.
- Inform the client that they may feel tired during the 24 hours following the class. Tiredness is not an unusual response to any deep bodywork. Please encourage them to drink more water to assist their body's change. Invited clients to contact you if they feel any discomfort or pain during the first 24 hours.
- As the client leaves, check they took their belongings and show them to the door.

You can now complete notes about the class and record the exercises. Write down any observations about the client's movement ability.

Returning clients

For a returning client, the key steps are:

- studio welcome
- workout
- booking review
- record attendance and payment
- farewell
- write up workout notes

Teaching online

Using technology as part of Pilates class offers is another way of supporting clients movement needs when they can't come to the studio. Pilates teachers, studio owners, and clients are now more open to online classes. Services like online recorded classes or live sessions are now also more available. Setting up these classes is still daunting for many teachers. It is not unreasonable for clients and teachers alike to have some concerns.

Client concerns may include:

- Staying safe and protected while working online.
- Maintaining their exercise routine even when they cannot access the studio.
- May not be sure what the benefits are of adding an online option.

Studio owner concerns may include:

- How to set up classes and the equipment needed to teach online
- What to charge
- How to communicate this new offer to their clients
- How to keep clients safe online

With a bit of planning and a few preparatory steps, you can set yourself up with a virtual studio. Below are some tips to help you become comfortable with online classes. It doesn't have to be perfect right from the start. You can make changes as you go along.

1. What are your studio needs?

Here are a few questions to help you decide what type of online services suit your studio best.

- Do you want to offer one-on-one, duet or small group sessions?
- Do you want to offer pre-recorded or live stream classes?
- Do you need to see all participants during the class?
- Do you have an online payment and scheduling method in place?

Once you have decided what your services will be, you can look at the different platforms. Zoom, Facetime, FB Messenger, Skype, and WhatsApp are all easy to set up and use. You need a device that connects to the internet. You can use your desktop computer, tablet or your phone. Using two devices, you can show the exercises from different angles. Charge up the old phone you had lying in a drawer; it doesn't have to be new and expensive. It just needs to have a good enough camera.

If your internet is choppy, you can connect an ethernet cable between your device and the router. Your clients can do the same to help keep their video from freezing and glitching.

When teaching Pilates classes, your sound is critical. Computer microphones are not of the best quality. Even a cheap microphone is a good investment. You do not need to spend a heap of money on improving your sound. Options for microphones include:

- lapel microphones
- ear pods
- free-standing microphones

Improving your sound quality

Make sure that whatever microphone you buy is compatible with your device. If you need music as part of your class, use a separate device to play the music. If you use a device with a built-in microphone and an external mic, you need to consider managing feedback. Most devices have sensitive microphones. But this sensitivity can also pick up ambient sounds from a busy or noisy environment. If the volume is too high, the microphone might pick up sounds from your speakers, creating a lasting echo effect.

So, if you're using an external microphone and get these annoying sounds, try moving it further away from your device speakers. You can also try lowering the speaker volume to reduce microphone pickup. You can test this by turning the volume down and increasing it a little at a time until you get an audible echo. Then reduce the volume back a notch and two, and you'll be back to fantastic clarity.

You can also use headphones or enable earbuds on your headset. Your volume output from your device will be completely isolated from the microphone.

You don't have to have perfect sound. But, make sure your sound is as straightforward as possible. Ask all participants to mute themselves to get rid of random noises. It will help not disturb other participants in your class.

Use tripods

You can use your phone, tablet or laptop to record or Livestream your classes. Using tripods for your devices makes life a lot easier. Once you have a good angle, put three squares of tape under the tripod legs so that you can set up with ease next time. If you want to zoom out, you can consider using your reformer carriage as a dolly. Remove the springs so you can pull the Reformer carriage back to widen the shot. Move it closer to tighten the frame. Keep the movement slow and steady.

Don't let this daunt you. Start the process. You can tweak it as you go along.

2. Staying safe when working online

You can help your clients stay safe when working online. If your online system allows, you can prevent this by implementing the following:

- adding a password
- turning off screen share for participants
- use a waiting room feature
- disable file transfer and join before host ability

Pre-recorded classes

If you choose to offer pre-recorded classes, you can use platforms like Youtube or Vimeo.

Youtube will let you save your videos and share them with your clients. You can upload a pre-recorded video. Set the video to be "Unlisted". Only people who have the link will be able to view the video. The cost for this is free, and you can share the video link with anyone.

A platform like Vimeo premium is more expensive. It is worth it if you want to take your entire business online. It lets you:

- live stream unlimited events
- embed the video player on your website
- brand the video player
- upload videos to your Vimeo channel.

Online membership sites give you flexibility as a teacher. You can also add another income stream to your business. You are also not limited by your geographical location.

There are many other options out there. Do your research and choose the business model and online hosting options that suit you best.

3.Booking and payment

An online booking and payment system will help manage communication with clients. They can schedule live class attendance and make payments without fuss. It takes a little to get it set up initially but it is worth it in the long run. The booking system can send out class reminders and keep track of their payment.

If you are setting up a membership option with pre-recorded videos, you will need to set up a recurring payment system and easily allow people to end their subscriptions.

4.Communicating with your clients

Create some socialising time

One of the main reasons people attend classes in person is to connect with others. You can create this with online classes too. Make some time available before the class for participants to chat.

You can also set up a community question and answer time where people can ask:

- about how their bodies work
- how to do specific exercises
- how to change positions to make an exercise easier
- exercises to suit their individual needs

Draw up a plan for your clients

Once you decide what works best for you and your clients, it's time to get your clients ready for this new option.

Tell your clients about the benefits.

Clients need to understand adding online classes is a good option for them. You can tell them about the importance of staying active and keeping moving between in-person classes. They may also travel for work. An online class option means they can continue to take care of their movement needs while travelling. Adding this option for clients can be another powerful motivator to sign up. By adding some extra value to your offer, you can make it even more appealing. Try promoting a unique four-week Pilates challenge. You can also add more value by creating an e-mail campaign or social media. Share a daily task or motivational tip with them every day. For example, walk somewhere in nature, or send them a new healthy recipe. These extra features can make it fun and exciting for them, regardless of whether you Livestream classes or publish recordings.

2. You will also need to let your clients know how to use your chosen online platform. If they need to create an account, give them specific details on doing this. Set up a selection of online class options on your schedule. You can offer these timeslots to your clients and add more as you go along. Let them know how you will communicate with them and give them the links they need to participate.

Technical and prop requirements

Give your clients all the information they need for their technical setup. You should also provide them with a list of props they need to do the exercises. You can share a link of where they can buy their props, or you can order and sell them to your clients. Help your clients understand what you need from them when they attend classes. Ask clients to:

- make sure they have a device with a big enough screen to see you for movement clarification
- check they have a stable internet connection. Use an ethernet cable if internet signals are patchy
- clear an ample space to move their arms and legs, so they don›t knock into anything
- set their mat, Reformer or other equipment up on a slight angle to the camera.
- place smaller pieces of equipment above their head end, so it stays out of the way when they move
- switch the camera off if they do not want corrections or to show themselves on camera
- switch their microphones to mute so any noise from their side does not disrupt everyone else.

Pricing

Keep your class prices the same. Your time and operational costs of the studio do not change. If you add a membership model to your existing studio business, add extra value to your offer to make it more attractive.

Tips for effective teaching online

- You may need to use more demonstration than in-person classes
- Setting your mat or equipment on diagonal and good lighting is essential.
- Wear solid coloured clothing. Avoid dark colours like black or charcoal grey. They can blend into the mat or upholstery. It makes it hard to see

the movements you are demonstrating.

- Avoid crazy patterns on your clothing too. It can distort the image on camera.
- Cue self-touch to help clients find alignment and become familiar with movements
- Check that your sound quality is clear and mute the participants when teaching. Unmute them when you need to ask any questions. If it is a yes or no answer, ask them to use a thumbs up or thumbs down sign with their hands
- Smiling while you teach improves your voice quality and makes you more approachable on camera.

CHAPTER 6 CLASSES

How to create great Pilates classes

Energy vs Time

M ost of us respond to rising demands in the studio by putting in longer hours. A lack of energy takes a toll on us in all areas of life. We experience a sense of overwhelm that leads to declining levels of engagement. We may also experience increased levels of distraction and even medical costs.

The core problem with working longer hours is that time is a finite resource. We need to prioritize our energy levels over how many hours we work.

To recharge your energy, you need to recognize the costs of energy-depleting behaviours. Then take responsibility for changing them for something better.

Establish rituals

Establishing simple rituals like these can lead to striking results. Inadequate nutrition, exercise, and sleep diminish your basic energy levels. You may also find your ability to manage emotions and focus your attention is harder to manage.

Identify rituals that help you build and renew your physical energy. When you take intermittent breaks for renewal, you will find more energy to reach your goals. The length of a renewal break is less important than the quality.

Manage your emotions

Take control of your emotions. Balancing your feelings helps you manage the external pressures you face better. To do this, become more aware of how you feel at various points during the day. Become aware of the impact emotions have on your effectiveness across your life.

Tip to defuse your negative emotions

Take the time to breathe in and out through your nose while noticing things around you. Only focus on what you can see. Name them -

plant, window, chair, desk etc. If that does not work for you, think of all the things that make you feel grateful. We can cultivate positive energy by learning to change the stories we tell ourselves about the events in our lives. Tell yourself the most hopeful stories possible.

How to plan your schedule for work-life balance

When I moved cities recently, I decided to set up my teaching time around the activities that gave me joy. I wrote down everything I wanted to do that made me smile and feel happy. Then I set up my schedule around these activities.

I scheduled my renewal time first! That does not mean I don't love what I do for my work life. I do. But, I tend always to put myself last and then over-stretch myself. When I do that, I start finding everything in life that bit too hard. I get grumpy.

My next step was to work out how many hours I wanted to teach each week. I calculated how many hours a week I felt I could give all my clients the energy and focus they deserved. Then I looked at my outgoings before calculating my potential earnings based on those hours. I found that I could earn more than I thought and have the life I wanted. You may need to make some adjustments to meet your needs but it is possible to make room in your life for everything that matters to you.

Setting up your classes

Teaching a group movement class is both challenging and rewarding. These classes give you a chance to be creative and have fun. Moving with other like-minded people is energising. A fun, upbeat group class can motivate people, so they want to come to more classes each week. Motivation to attend classes means they will see physical improvement. The more progress they make, the more they will gain a sense of satisfaction. When presenting a group workout, there are six steps to keep in mind:

- Teach to your strength

- Accommodate different learning styles
- Use simple language
- Choose a focus for your class
- Provide an introductory series to teach clients correct body positions and machine interaction
- Set multi-level exercise options

Teach to your strengths

If you are a runner, cyclist or golfer, you may want to consider creating a sport-specific class. Focussing on a particular sport can help people achieve their sporting goals. It can help clients to balance their training schedule. Or, you can teach them to use muscles differently to be more resilient and reduce the risk of injury. Know the history of each client before you teach them.

Cue for different learning styles

To connect with everyone in the group, you need to cue for all learners. Use a variety of cues throughout your class. Think of cues that may resonate with visual, auditory and kinaesthetic learners. Developing this skill keeps the class moving and help you include everyone.

Safety first

Always cue for safety as soon as you see something going amiss. Look out for changes in alignment that could cause an injury. Check spring settings and straps before they do the exercise.

Examples of cueing for different learning styles

Visual: Use demonstration when necessary on your own body or someone else's. Use imagery cues to create a picture of what they are trying to achieve in the clients' minds.

Auditory: Use a sound such as a hissing exhalation or "aaaah" at an appropriate point in the exercise. Sound cues may help clients stabilise their bodies.

Tactile: Cue self-touch to help people orientate their body awareness. If their shoulders get tense, ask them to tap the top of the shoulders and do a few shoulder shrugs.

Combine your cues

A tactile cue with imagery or auditory cue can further help your clients. They can connect with the exercise or body alignment change.

Use simple language

Be consistent in your language use when communicating with your clients. Try and avoid using medical-sounding terms as they can cause clients to feel confused. Your classes can learn new concepts over time, but you need to factor in time to explain these concepts to them. Don't expect them to remember everything in only one class. Repeat and expand on the information over successive classes.

Choose a focus for your class

Having a focus for your class helps you make good exercise choices. A theme can also help you to create classes that flow well. For example, you could choose to focus on spinal mobility. Then direct your cues to achieve a more in-depth understanding of this. You don't neglect the other body areas; they don't feature as much. You still want to build a positive, fun full-body movement experience with every class. But you can help clients understand how their spine moves. You can also create an awareness of how their limbs can amplify the work of their spine. You can support them to either reduce or increase the range of motion in the spine. Then you can apply this new knowledge to an everyday movement like walking.

Set multi-level exercise options

Instructors will need to teach a multi-option class. You will give options for props, body positions and ranges of movement. Start by providing the simple option first for 2-3 repetitions. Then offer the next option. Each variation should build on the previous one.

Establish beginner classes

As a studio owner, you will need to set out a pathway for new clients. You also need to help teachers to be effective communicators. We all teach uniquely. Clients get used to the way we express ourselves. Each time you work with a new teacher, it takes time to become familiar with how they explain exercises. New clients must fulfil your criteria, regardless of how many classes they have attended in the past.

In some cases, new clients may need to attend private classes first. They can then develop the skills they need to succeed in a group class. Preparing clients to enter into a group-training situation requires them to:

- Understand how to breathe well and use breathe while moving
- Establish and maintain alignment while moving
- Be familiar with a range of baseline exercises
- Be able to choose a position or modification of an exercise appropriate to them.

Class structure - Mat, Reformer, Studio privates and semi-privates

In an ideal world, timetabled classes based on clients' level of competence is best. An introductory package can help clients build up knowledge over time. It allows them to assimilate good movement skills. After that, clients can attend the next level class with a good basic understanding. But this structured setup is not always possible. Some exercise environments make classes available without managing ability levels. Sometimes people with different levels of ability and experience attend the same class. Multi-level classes bring another level of challenge to teaching classes.

Mixed level classes work best when progressing exercises from simple to more complex. Start with an essential movement skill and then move through different levels. Ask class participants to identify the level that is right for them. If they progress and feel the exercise is too strenuous, they can do the previous version. Create a safe environment where clients take responsibility for making good movement choices.

In a mixed class, beginners can focus on an introductory movement. This same exercise gives more experienced participants a way to warm up. They can then progress to a more challenging repertoire. Often, 'perfecting' a simple movement can be more difficult.

Mastering basic movements help when the exercise becomes more difficult. Clients will have more focus, strength and stability to perform the movements better. It is always good to get back to basics.

Props are also helpful when addressing different abilities in the class. Advanced clients can decrease the resistance level of an exercise. They will need to focus more on controlling the movement. A beginner can gain more help by increasing the resistance, making the exercise easier for them. They can concentrate on achieving correct form without risking injury.

Use gentle encouragement throughout the class. You can boost the client's confidence to keep improving. You can motivate clients through specific praise and exercise progressions.

Five ways to modify exercises

A modification is when you simplify an exercise. It is an exercise variation if you find ways to increase the challenge.

- Simplify the exercise

Many exercises are complex. Clients may struggle to perform the exercise well. Break the exercise into component pieces. Teach each section before combining them and practising the entire movement.

- Shorten the levers

Your arms and legs can act as levers. You use them to place resistance at the point furthest away (distal) from the body. If a client cannot remain stable, it would be better to reduce the resistance. For example, ask them to bend their legs or place their forearms on the floor.

- Increase help/decrease resistance

Sometimes adding more resistance can help a client to perform an exercise better. To decrease the resistance, reduce the weight they are working against. A lighter resistance can make an exercise more challenging. It means the client has to find more control. If the resistance is too heavy, they will change their alignment. They may work too hard to achieve the exercise, resulting in injury. They are not yet strong enough to work against the higher resistance.

- Props

Any tool that helps the client with an exercise is a prop. Props can assist the client in achieving the desired result or adding an extra challenge to the exercise. Placing a folded towel under a clients head to adjust their alignment is an example of a prop. Add a flex ring or foam roller to assist or challenge clients.

- Speed

Speed is both a modification and variation tool. Slowing the pace can assist a client in following the flow of a movement sequence. It can also be challenging to do specific exercises at a slower pace. It is important never to sacrifice the rhythm or flow of an exercise when playing with speed.

Nine ways to progress exercises

The suggestions below are by no means the only way to approach progressing a client. Your clients' individual needs, goals and learning styles will guide this process. It is helpful to have a framework to follow. Switch the steps below if necessary. You do not need to follow the steps in precisely the order given.

Help your clients to take responsibility for their movement journey. Relate the movements they do in class to everyday life whenever you can. That way, you can give them tools to apply to everyday life situations. Below are some ideas to explore.

1. Start with alignment and breathing

Start by explaining why alignment and breathing are important to be aware of. Give your clients different ways to experience these concepts. These tools can help them breathe and bring awareness to poor alignment choices. I like to start alignment exploration by getting my clients to dance. I learned this technique from an Alexander practitioner. It is powerful and simple for anyone to use. We choose a piece of music that gets the clients' toes tapping and dancing together. Dancing feels silly at the beginning. But, it breaks the ice, elevates their mood and makes them less self-conscious as the song progresses. I then ask them to reduce the movement until they do an invisible dance. When they feel tense or *'stuck'* in their body, they can do the invisible dance. Or, they can choose to put on a piece of music and dance away.

2. Create awareness

Awareness helps clients identify their poor postural habits so they can change the way they stand, sit, and walk. Once they are more aware of how they move, you can ask them to link an exercise to this pattern. For example, when they stand up out of the chair with poor mechanics, ask them to focus on using the tools you shared with them to improve their movements. They then repeat it three times before going where they intended. If a client wants to improve their balance, They can stand on one leg and brush their teeth. Linking movements to everyday life situations means saving time and making a change. It also means they will get more out of their time with you in the studio.

Using benchmarking to increase awareness and proprioception

Benchmarking gives clients time to build an image of how their body has changed. Their brain can make connections between exercises and positive outcomes. Identifying a positive result will motivate them to do the exercise again. They are less likely to need your supervision each time. They are more likely to take ownership of their well-being.

You will need to help them make sense of their experience in the beginning. We are not used to qualifying what our bodies experience beyond pleasure or pain. With pain, we often overlook it and go on regardless. It is an annoyance rather than something to explore. Clients may notice a change but lack the words. Ask them some questions and give them options. 'Does your leg feel longer or shorter on the side we worked?' If they can›t find the words, I may say, ‹To me, it looks like that leg is longer. What do you think?›

Over time they start to volunteer their experience without you asking. It is a signal that clients are taking ownership of their inner experience. It is very cool to observe this change.

How to use benchmarking

After doing an exercise on one side. Close your eyes and take some time to become aware of your body. Compare the two sides. Take note of any differences you feel. For example,

- o Do both shoulders feel like they are sitting level? Or is one higher than the other?
- o Do your legs feel the same length?

Don't judge what you find. Please note the differences and store them in the back of your mind or write them down. Take some time to assess what has changed in your body? Do you feel more length more flexibility? Again store the information. Repeat the exercise on the other side and then benchmark again.

3. Dynamic movements

Add some small dynamic movements that help to explain the way a particular joint or body area works. You can then use benchmarking again. Then progress to a more significant movement. Build on what they learned from the essential exercise.

4. Add load

Many Pilates exercises start lying on the floor on your back. Quadruped positions and movements are suitable to progress and introduce increased load. Check that the client has no knee or wrist conditions,

82

making this a poor choice. The appropriate load progression in exercises classes is complex. There are many factors to consider, such as, fear, pain, degree of healing from an injury/surgery or an inflammatory response. If you feel out of your depth, seek professional medical help. Refer your client to an appropriate person like a physiotherapist. They can help you with the proper degree of load and guide you through the stages to recovery. This collaboration will ensure your client is safe and the programme is successful.

5. Change the position

Look for ways to change the position to make moves slightly different. For example, do supine arm movements on the mat and then progress to a quadruped position. Apply the knowledge from the more supported work to the more challenging one.

6. Change the type of resistance

Movements will always feel different when you change the resistance. Change from using the springs used with the Pilates equipment to resistance bands. This change offers various ways to work your muscles.

7. Go from two legs/arms to one leg/arm

One of the most exciting ways to change exercises is to use only one arm or one leg at a time. Clients need more coordination and can improve balance control too.

8. Add a balance challenge

Even more challenging than unilateral exercises is using something unstable. You can use a ball, foam roller, trampoline or inflatable disc. Make it more difficult if it is safe to do by asking clients to close their eyes.

9. Do more compound movements

Two exercises at once can save time and add a new dimension to your exercise choices. For example, try balancing on one leg as you perform a rotator cuff strengthening exercise.

Class plan

You can divide your class into roughly six (6) sections. The warm-up, full-body integration and cool down are always in the same place in your lesson. You can shuffle each of the remaining areas around as you need to to make the class flow.

You can also add elements of each area into the others to help keep classes fun and give a sense of variety. The six sections of a class consist of:

- warm-up
- abdominals
- rib cage, arms, shoulders, and legs
- spinal motion
- integration
- cool down.

Decide on a focus for the class ahead of time. You can choose anything such as breathing, improving arm strength or balance control. You can also choose to work toward a specific exercise. Be creative and do exercises that lead to this specific one. It is not always necessary for you to announce the focus to the class, but it gives you a framework on which to base your class. These themes will also become more evident as you work with a group over time. You will observe where clients are struggling over time. Then you can design classes to help them achieve their goals.

Always check that you don't add too many changes of position. Try and design your class, so you move to a different position and do what you need to do there before changing. Flopping from your back, tummy, sitting, and then lying down again can make a class feel disjointed. Consider how your class will flow.

PLEASE NOTE: The times listed next to each section are an approximate guide only. It should help you with pacing in the beginning. But, do not rush if you find that you are getting short of time. Instead, try and change your list of chosen exercises. Leave out some that don't help you achieve your goal. It is more important that you clarify points to your clients. Don't worry about the content if something comes up that needs more attention. Focus on giving them a great movement experience. They don't know what you planned. Save it for the next class.

Warm-up (10-15 minutes)

Our feet are essential for quality of life. Starting a class by grounding people is very powerful. Sore, stiff, inflexible feet stop people from moving. Sore feet impact people's quality of life. Spending a few minutes at the start of class on releasing the feet will help alignment and stability. The warm-up should contain the most necessary basic building block exercises. A warm-up will prepare your clients for more complex movements to come. When working on your class plan, this is the last step. You need to know all the exercises you are focussing on during your class. Then you can decide on appropriate pre-Pilates exercises for the warm-up.

Abdominals (5 minutes)

Blend shoulder stabilisation into abdominals at the end of the warm-up to create a bridge from simple to more complex movements. You can also add some of the hip alignment and activation work into your abdominal sequencing.

Rib cage, arms, shoulders and legs (20-25 min)

You can start adding some load and resistance at this stage of the class. Expand on the warm-up—Challenge clients with various controlled and dynamic movements. Or focus on creating joint range of motion if they lack flexibility. Make them aware of the functional nature of these exercises as you teach, such as using hip hinges to get in and out of a chair without loading their spines. Relate these sit-to-stand actions to the exercise *Bridge with Leg Up*. Or relate the hip strengthening work to climbing stairs, walking or running. *Sidekick* is an excellent example of an exercise that teaches these skills.

Spinal motion (10 minutes)

If you have already done abdominal work, you have started moving the spine into flexion. Include extension, rotation and side flexion in a variety of ways. Your aim should always be to give clients a balanced programme so they can feel strong and supple when they leave the class.

Integration (5-10 minutes)

Choose a more complex exercise. You can then apply many of the previous learning experiences in the class. Clients can learn to build their skill level and combine what they have learned already. You will need to reference the exercises they did during the class already. Then help clients to apply this knowledge and perform the exercise with success.

Cooldown (5 minutes)

You can use spinal motion movements you may not have worked on yet, such as side flexion, to transition into this part of the class. You can also do targeted stretching exercises. Focus on the body parts that had a heavy strengthening focus during the class. Stretching is a good option for evening classes. Avoid prolonged end range stretching during the day. They could be more prone to injury if they do more strenuous activities after attending your class.

Creating flow

Creating flow in your classes

Teaching Pilates is both a science and an art. 'Flow' is one of the ten principles of the Pilates method. Introducing flow in your group classes relies on:

1. exercise selection
2. clear transitions between exercises.

What exactly is flow?

You can think of flow as creating ways to transition from one exercise to another. These transitions should make the class continuous, smooth and elegant. Archetypal postures offer a variety of options to transition between exercises.

Benefits of adding flow

1. Save time: Transitions helps you sequence your class. Clients will feel like they are getting more exercise time and better value for money. Stop-starting isn't wrong or bad. But it does waste a lot of time. Making your transitions count opens up more options for creativity in your classes.
2. Increases challenge: When you incorporate flow, your clients will feel more challenged. You don›t need to add challenging exercises. Using flow in your class will help keep clients moving and help cut downtime.
3. Beats exercise boredom The main reason people stop their exercise programme is boredom. By using a variety of class formats, you will motivate your clients and keep them engaged.
4. Fun, social interactions Moving with others is inspiring. Sharing time with people who enjoy the same activity as you do as an adult helps you feel connected. It builds camaraderie among participants and the instructor.

Self-evaluation

Teaching, like learning, is a continuous process. It has no beginning, middle or end. As teachers, we work alone, even in a busy studio. To stay motivated, it helps if we can check our teaching. There are three aspects to the teaching cycle:

1. planning
2. implementing
3. evaluating

These three aspects of teaching interweave. We often don't realise that we cycle through them in many ways all the time. Effective teaching requires us to use all three phases of the cycle.

Planning

Planning involves developing learning objectives:

1. designing the method to achieve the objectives
2. deciding on the assessment
3. take time to decide if we have reached our goal for the class

You will generally have a plan prepared when you walk into the studio. There is no set way to design your plan. You could begin with the goal and move to the method. Other times you may have an assessment, and it will help you determine the intent and strategy you will use. Or, you find a great activity to plan a class around.

An experienced teacher may have the plan laid out in their head. At the same time, a new teacher may need to write it down. Whatever form the lesson plan is in, it is the backbone of good teaching!

Implementation

The implementation of the plan involves putting the plan into action. Success often rests with your ability to manage clients and the studio environment.

Motivation is instrumental in the success of the session. Every client will have a different motivating factor. For some clients, it could be:

- reducing pain and discomfort
- aesthetic purposes
- time for themselves
- meeting other people who love to move
- curiosity about Pilates
- fun activity to join

Whatever the reason, clients need a reason to become engaged in physical activity. Motivating your clients is a crucial factor in becoming successful as a teacher. Experienced teachers have learned good motivation techniques. They have also learned that different things encourage different clients. They know how to use this knowledge as they teach.

Evaluation

Taking the time to evaluate your teaching is vital to your success. This activity allows you to discover the worth of your work and is a subjective process.

It is a process that must consider many factors, and this is no easy task as each client is different. The environment in which people learn is vital to the evaluation process. To remain motivated, you must find value in what you do. Most jobs have some measure of success. You need to find your measure.

Made in United States
Troutdale, OR
12/05/2024

25890584R00060